Power Bodybuilding

Program Structure

This is a high frequency, dual-focused training program where myofibrillar and sarcoplasmic hypertrophy are both targeted over two phases; a strength phase where progressive overload is the primary focus, and a hypertrophy phase where strength progression is tempered with hypertrophy-focused progression. The body is trained over 3 workouts, which each workout placing its focus on those two aspects of muscle growth— increasing contractile strength through progressive overload and increasing non-contractile growth through increased blood flow and nutrient partitioning. The routine is meant to be performed exactly as listed. Movements are to be performed in the order listed. There is enough allowed variation in the "additional movements" and set number/methods to keep the routine feeling fresh for the duration of the program.

This program alternates 6-week overload cycles with a 1-week "de-load" period in between each phase. Thus, a single rotation through the complete program is a 14-week endeavor. This can be adjusted as needed for each individual person. Since the limiting factor to progression and results will be one's ability to continue improving in strength for the movements being used, a strength plateau indicates that progress with this program will be stalled. If a strength plateau is reached and progress begins to stall, it is recommended that a short "de-load" is taken where the user backs off on the intensity and workload for as long as necessary before restarting the program with the same core structure. As phase 1 of the program places more emphasis on pure strength progression, an optional extra "de-load" day is included on each 8-day progression through the training cycle. If any day of the training cycle results in zero new PRs set, then it is recommended that this 9th day is taken to recover before restarting the training cycle. Since phase 2 of the program is more hypertrophy focused, there tends to be less need for additional de-load days. In phase 2, if the user completes a full workout without a single PR, it is recommended that an additional day off is taken in that training cycle as well.

Program Focus

The focus of phase 1 in this program is increasing muscular size through progressively overloading the muscle to force myofibrillar adaptation to an ever-increasing load. This strength adaptation essentially falls into two primary categories.

1. **Getting stronger in a movement.** This means that you're able to lift more weight in an exercise—this is essentially powerlifting. There is NOT a one-to-one correlation to getting stronger in a movement and increased muscle mass in the muscles used for that movement. Getting stronger in a movement

can occur because of improved mechanical advantage, neurological adaptation, better supporting equipment, variations in diet, rest time between sets, and location of the movement in the workout (first exercises vs last exercise). While our focus IS getting stronger in the exercises we perform, the goal isn't simply to move more weight in a movement—it's to increase the strength of the intended muscle.

2. **Making a muscle stronger.** This means that the muscles performing the movement are getting stronger—not just that you are able to move a heavier bar from point A to point B. This type of strength increase is slower and less obvious. This type of strength is also much more closely correlated to myofibrillar hypertrophy—or the actual growth of contractile tissue. Phase 1 of this program focuses on this version of muscular adaptation. Ultimately—to be a powerlifting bodybuilder, you must have very strong muscles (which will also be large). If you were to decide to compete in powerlifting, specialization training on improving your biomechanical advantage and neurological adaptation can become a central focus to perform better in a meet—but I must stress that these adaptations do not mean a stronger muscle and don't correlate to a bigger muscle tissue.

Phase 2 in this program moves its focus more intently on purely hypertophic adaptation. There remains a strong sub-focus on increasing the strength of the worked muscle, but only in the manner that an increase in contractile strength leads to an increase in muscle size. Each workout places some focus on progressive overload as well as some focus on sarcoplasmic growth—or "blood volume" training. The way in which phase 2 of the program tracks progress and looks for growth is as follows:

3. **Making a muscle stronger.**
   This means that the muscles performing the movement are getting stronger—not that you have become more biomechanically efficient in the movement. There is a difference between getting stronger in a movement and making a muscle stronger. Getting stronger in a movement can occur because of improved mechanical advantage, neurological adaptation, better supporting equipment, variations in diet, rest time between sets, and location of the movement in the workout (first exercises vs last exercise). Getting stronger because of a stronger muscle means that no outside changes have occurred that would improve your strength in a movement. The same form is used, the same machine is used, the same rest period is used, etc. This type of strength increase is MUCH slower and less obvious than simply getting stronger in a movement. However, it is MUCH more closely correlated to an increase in muscle

size. A stronger contractile tissue is largely the result of an increase in muscle proteins that make up the contractile tissue of the muscle.

4. **Making a muscle's sub-components larger.** This doesn't necessarily mean that we are always focused on setting PRs in every exercise. There is some aspect to training that is unrelated to muscular strength but increases the size of a muscle. It is hard to argue that there isn't some benefit to non-strength increasing training that focuses on increasing blood flow to the trained muscle, looks to increase the "pump" of that muscle, and likely produces as much or more DOMS as the training that focuses on making a muscle stronger.

Program Structure – Phase 1

All red colored sets are "PR sets" or "myofibrillar sets." Your primary focus in these sets is hitting a PR without any change to form, rest time, or any other variable other than muscular strength. You MUST hit at least one PR in the "core" movement (squats, bench, deadlifts) every single workout. You SHOULD hit at least one PR for every single body part. You should TRY to hit a PR in every red colored set of every workout.

Program Structure – Phase 2

Phase 2 continues with the red colored "PR sets," but includes a higher number of black colored sets than phase 1. In phase 2, these black colored sets are considered "hypertrophy sets" or "sarcoplasmic sets" where the goal isn't necessarily to get stronger, but rather to bring blood flow to the tissues and get as good of a "pump" as possible to emphasize sarcoplasmic adaptations. Strength increases in these sets will be happily accepted, but that is not the primary goal of the sets.

Day-to-Day Focus

While the general approach to both phases in this protocol is progressive overload, there are multiple adaptations in which a muscle group grows larger. If you were to slice through the cross-sectional area of a muscle group in half, you would see that the majority of the "muscle" is not contractile tissue, but instead a conglomerate of fluid volume, blood vessels, capillary density, and other non-protein components. While increasing the contractile strength of the associated proteins will indirectly increase the size of these components as well, there is a more direct approach to stimulating the growth of the non-contractile muscle components. This is where the daily workout programming becomes important.

How can we maximize training frequency without the risk of over training and injury? Clearly there is a point where a muscle can be trained—and trained relatively intensely—without a physiological level of DOMs. This is the key to increasing the frequency of training, maximizing the rate of strength increases, and stimulating the maximum amount of muscle protein synthesis.

How is this approached?

1. The part of training that the "bro-split" gets correct is the need for increased blood flow to the trained tissues and the delayed onset muscle soreness associated with high intensity, higher volume training. Training frequency can be maximized if muscle soreness is minimized—but that does not also optimize the synthesis of new muscle tissue— it only maximizes the number of times in which a PR can be attempted. There is some benefit to the increased volume that comes with training a body part to the point of noticeable soreness.
2. The part of training that the "bro-split" gets incorrect is that most people, if they're training reasonably hard under a reasonably high workload, they're probably creating a stimulus for new protein synthesis that is higher than their recovery and diet can cover. If this were not the case, then for any given training program, an increase in training volume should create a correlating increase in muscle growth—but this isn't the case. This is also the explanation for why so many top bodybuilders seem to be able to train with limited

intensity while still growing—because most people are training harder than they can locally (locally as in the short term) cover completely through diet and rest.

How do we correct for these issues?

1. Focus some effort of each training session on maximizing the sarcoplasmic aspects of hypertrophy. This means that some body parts of each training day will need to be trained to the point of soreness.
2. Focus some effort of each training session on maximizing strength/PR progression without taxing recovery to the point of those muscle groups seeing DOMs to any appreciable level.

Types of Muscle Growth

Myofibrillar Hypertrophy

The standard understanding of muscle growth is that the myosin and actin contractile fibers increase in size and number through the synthesis of new proteins. This results in an increase in muscular strength and an increase in muscle size. The idea that this is the only form of muscle growth is a hot topic in the science of muscle building. The problem with the idea of myofibrillar growth being the only form of muscle growth is that it does nothing to explain the vast differences in muscle size between professional bodybuilders and competitive weightlifters. In addition, anyone who's ever seen a piece of steak can quickly spot the difference between a fresh cut of meat and one that has been dried into beef jerky. If all that remains once a cut of meat is dried out is the actual contractile proteins of the meat, then what is all that other stuff? Steak is made of muscle—are we to believe that the only portion of that muscle which can be influenced through weight training is that small portion that remains as beef jerky?

Myofibrillar hypertrophy is still the primary focus of this training program. Regardless of whether there are other forms of hypertrophy, the fact that a stronger tissue will be a more resilient tissue and will likely amply the ability for any other types of hypertrophy to occur remains true. Training a muscle under a heavy load in the rep range and time under tension that appears to stimulate protein synthesis most effectively will work—new proteins will be synthesized to the myosin and actin and the result will be a larger, stronger muscle tissue. This is where our PR focused training comes into play.

Sarcoplasmic Hypertrophy

The idea of a non-myofibrillar form of hypertrophy is becoming more accepted in the science community. If you look at it from a logical standpoint, it seems hard to wave off the size discrepancy between athletes like Olympic weightlifters—who are incredibly strong and explosive with that of professional bodybuilders—who have a greatly reduced strength level but much larger muscle mass as just normal variance. Something is clearly different—whether the difference in size is called "muscle" is really just a semantic argument. The cross-sectional area of a bodybuilder's muscle is much larger than that of athletes who are much stronger. You could argue that the non-contractile portion of that cross-sectional area isn't technically muscle mass, but if it increases the volume of the muscle and appears to be influenced by training, then I don't see why it matters what you call it. It can be increased through training and it increases the size of the muscle—period.

Training for each Type of Growth

Myofibrillar Training

As I said above—the point of the myofibrillar portion of the training is to create stronger muscles. This is done by *progressive overload* and breaking PRs in your training sessions.

So, what constitutes a PR? At its core, it's using either more weight for the same number of reps or doing more reps with the same number of weight, but there is more to it than that.

This thought process is where people FAIL in progressive overload.

We aren't simply trying to get stronger in a movement (this isn't powerlifting). We're trying to make a MUSCLE stronger. If you did 10 reps with 405 on squats last week and 11 reps this week—BUT to get those 11 reps you widened your stance for better leverage, then *you didn't make the muscle stronger*. You simply found a better mechanical advantage.

Set variations that do not count as a PR

- Changing your form.
  - Widening your stance on squats

- Placing the bar lower on your back
- Adjusting the seat to a more mechanically advantageous position on a machine
- Taking a longer rest period.
  - If you get a PR because you rested an extra minute between sets, you were just more rested—not stronger. Taking 10 minutes between sets isn't bodybuilding
- Changing machines.
  - A PR set on a machine is for that machine only
- Changing the order of the workout.
  - If your previous PR on a back movement was with that movement as the third exercise, then moving that to the first exercise so the muscle is fresher is not a PR

Sarcoplasmic Training

The sarcoplasmic training portion of this program should be the most familiar to readers. It is essentially the standard type of training shown in nearly every bodybuilder's training program since the sport began. Although any chance to increase the weight used in a movement should be taken advantage of, the goal of this portion of the program isn't setting PRs. The goal in the sarcoplasmic training sets is to lift in the manner that current studies show to stimulate the greatest level of muscle protein synthesis following training.

Considerations for sarcoplasmic Growth

- Lift explosively. The concentric (positive) portion of the rep should be completed in rapid form. While you may have been taught that "good form" involves slow controlled reps, I urge you to consider the difference between "good form" and "form that builds muscle" because studies on the subject show that an explosive concentric motion is most effective

- Focus on getting a "pump" in the muscle. We're looking to increase blood flow to the tissue. We want the tissue to be overwhelmed with blood flow to the point that its only recourse is to increase the size and density of its blood vessels and capillary beds. These things take up space in the muscle tissue and increasing their size and density will add size to the tissue—as well as increasing the functional capacity of that tissue to bring and remove nutrients and waste products.

- It's not entirely clear what role delayed onset muscle soreness (DOMS) plays in muscle growth, but the fact that our sarcoplasmic training will include a higher number of sets and reps than the myofibrillar focused portions means that soreness will be higher in the muscles targeted with the sarcoplasmic training. Because of this, the workload of the program is structured such that which muscles will experience greater DOMS is taken into consideration.

Phase 1

6 weeks

Training Split – Phase 1

Day 1: Push

Day 2: Legs

Day 3: Pull 1

Day 4: off

Day 5: Push

Day 6: Legs

Day 7: Pull 2

Day 8: off

Day 9: optional off day

Push

Core Movements – Perform each week

Flat Barbell Bench Press
3-4 sets x 10-12 reps (building up in weight for the main set—take as many as needed.)
1 set 8-10 reps
3 set 5-7 reps

- Find a way to get PRs on this every week
- On the 3 sets of 5-7 reps, you have multiple ways of achieving a PR
    - You can increase the total number of reps over the three sets. For example, if you did 3 sets of 5 reps with a weight this week for a total of 15 reps, then 1 set of 6 reps and 2 sets of 5 reps with the same weight the following week would be a 16 rep PR
    - Increasing the weight you use. Once you hit 7 reps in all three sets, you can increase the weight used
    - Increase the weight on the first set, and then complete the second two sets with the same weight and reps as the previous week.

Hammer Strength Press (any version):
1 rest pause set of 11-15 reps total

- Stick with the same machine until you hit sticking point on PRs—then move to a different machine and do the same thing. Cycle through so you're always hitting a PR

Seated Military Press:

1 set 10-12 reps
1 set of 5-7 reps

- Perform as many warm up sets as needed

Seated Lateral Raises:

1 multiple drop set

- Start with a heavy dumbbell that you can get about 10 reps with. Hit 10 reps, then drop 5-10lbs in dumbbell weight and do another 10 reps, continue dropping until you're using only your arms

Close Grip Bench:

2 sets 8-10 reps

- Try to hit PRs, but make sure your triceps are doing the work—not your chest

Overhead Rope Extensions:

3 sets 15-20 reps

- These are done as a mechanical drop set. Start with hands separated. When you hit failure that way, keep hands separated on the eccentric, but put hands together (for leverage) on the positive portion. When you hit failure there, keep hands together the entire time and bang out a few extra partial reps

Pec Deck:

4 sets 20 reps

- Pure blood volume here—get blood in the area

Additional Movements – choose 1-2 movements per workout

Dips:
2 sets to failure

Clean and presses:
2 sets 12-15 reps (hang clean to press)

Replacement Movements – replace a core movement when you hit sticking point on PRs

Cable Crossovers:
4 sets 20 reps (as replacement for pec deck)

Incline Dumbbell Presses:
1 set x 8-10 reps (as flat barbell replacement)

Incline Barbell presses:
1 set x 8-10 reps (as flat barbell replacement)

Legs

Standing Calf (any variation):
4 sets x 15-20 reps

- Squeeze these—don't bounce. These aren't PR sets. Your goal is to contract the calf, not bounce up more weight

Seated Calf:
2-3 sets x 15-20 reps

- At the start of the movement, lean your body forward to place more weight over your feet. As the set gets harder, begin leaning back until you're actively pulling back on the handles to extend the set

Core Movements – perform every workout

Walking lunges:
3 sets 30 total steps (warm up)

Lying Leg curls:
2-4 warm up sets (warm up as long as needed)
1 set x 10-12 reps

- Add 1-2 forced reps, partial reps, and/or slow negative

Squat (back squat or front squat – rotate between them as needed to always hit a PR):
2-3 sets 10-20 reps (just a warm up—use as many sets and reps as needed but treat them as warm ups. They are not

to be anywhere near failure)

1 set x 6-8 reps

1 set x 20 reps

- You have two exercise options to use to hit a PR. You must hit a PR on at least one of the primary sets WITHOUT changing form or rest period between sets. If you know you're not going to hit a PR on either set on back squats this week, then switch to front squats and find a way to grind out either 21 reps with your previous best weight or move up in weight for 20 reps

Seated Leg Curls:

2 sets x 10-15 reps

- Your PR is the total reps with the same weight over the two sets (somewhere between 20-30 reps). A PR is more total reps than the previous workout

Leg extension – Sissy squat super set

1 sets of:

20 reps on leg extension

Failure on body weight sissy squats

- The leg extensions are to positive failure. The sissy squats should follow IMMEDIATELY (within 5 seconds) of finishing the leg extensions
- You should hate this. If you enjoy this, you're not working hard enough

Adductor Machine

1 set of 20 reps

- Look to increase weight on this every week—but make sure you're squeezing your adductors, not just getting a better biomechanical leverage

Additional movements – choose 1-2 movements each workout

Wide stance stiff leg deadlifts:
2-3 sets x 12-15 reps (a few reps short of failure)

Bulgarian split squats:
1 set x 20 reps per leg

Single Leg presses:
2 sets 15-20 reps

Hack Squats:
1 set 15-20 reps

Pull 1 - Back Thickness

Warm up:

- Do a few sets of pull downs or cable pull overs to get blood in the lats and muscles around the shoulder.

Core Movements -- Perform each week

Pull ups – Neutral Grip:

3 sets to failure

- Work on getting more reps per set each week. When you can complete 50 reps in three sets, begin adding weight to the movement by adding chains around your neck or putting a dumbbell between your feet.

Deadlifts, Rack Deads, or T-Bar Rows:

Warm ups: as many as needed to get to your max weight

1 set x 5-8 reps

1 set x 10-12 reps

- Just like on squats, you have more than one movement to work with. If you're feeling strong on deads, always use those as the primary movement. If your legs are too sore from the leg workout, use rack deads or T-bar rows as your back up movement.

Face Pulls:

3 sets x 10-12 reps

- This is essentially a pull-down to the face rather than to the chest. It focuses more on upper back than the lats.

Shrugs: (any variation)

4x15

Preacher curls:

1 rest pause set 15-20 reps

- Use as many warm ups as needed before the one all-out set

Drag Curls:

2 sets x 20 reps

- A PR is your 2 set total rep combination (about 40 reps). Get either more total reps or more weight each week.

Additional movements – choose 1-2 movements each workout

Seated Rows:

3 sets x 10-15 reps

- Same as usual—focus on getting stronger on these. Change grips each week

Hammer Strength pulldowns (any variation):

3 sets x 10-12

Hammer Strength Rows (any variation):

3 sets x 8-10 reps

Dumbbell rows (any variation):
2 sets x 15-20 reps

Cable curls (any variation):
6 sets 6 reps

- This is done one arm at a time—it's essentially one very long set where you rotate between arms for 6 sets of each arm. Only perform an additional bicep movement on EITHER the pull1 or pull 2 workouts—not both.

Pull 2 - Back Width

Warm up:

- Perform a few sets of cable pull overs or light pulldowns to get the muscles of the back and shoulder properly warm and ready for the training session

Core Movements – Perform each week

Pull downs (overhand grip):
2-3 sets x 10-12 reps (not to failure—increase weight each set)
1 set x 10-12 reps

- Focus on squeezing the lats. Pulldowns aren't a strength movement. Spread the scapula and then contract the lats. That is the goal here. If we can get stronger in that form—great. But don't sacrifice the contraction for weight.

Reverse grip pulldowns:
2-3 sets x 10-12 reps (not to failure)
1 set x 10-12 reps

- Same as over hand grip. The point is the squeeze the lats. If you can get stronger, great—but don't sacrifice form.

Way bent over rows:
2 sets x 10 reps
1 set x 20 reps

- Stand on a box if needed. These are bent over rows with a wider grip (a lot wider) where you stay bent over past parallel to the floor. You pull to the chest on these.

Barbell Curls:

1 Rest Pause set 15-20 total reps

- 1-2 warm up sets to get blood in the area and then right into the main set

Dumbbell Hammer Curls:

1 set 15-20 reps

- Straight set, not rest pause. Start with both arms at the same time. When you get close to failure, begin alternating arms for more momentum and leverage.

Additional movements – choose 1-2 movements each workout

Hammer Strength pulldowns (any variation):
3 sets x 10-12

Hammer Strength Rows (any variation):
3 sets x 8-10 reps

Machine Curls (any variation):
6 sets x 6 reps

- Perform an additional bicep movement on EITHER pull 1 or pull 2, not both. This is meant to alternate between arms, so it would be essentially one very long set where you do 6 reps back and forth between arms

Phase 2

6 weeks

Training Split – Phase 2

Day 1: Push 1

- Chest, Side Delt -- Hypertrophy focus
- Front Delt, Triceps -- PR focus

Day 2: Legs 1

- Quads, Calves -- Hypertrophy focus
- Hams, Adductors, Glutes -- PR focus

Day 3: Off

Day 4: Pull 1

- Lats, Rear Delts, Biceps -- Hypertrophy focus
- Mid/Lower Back, Traps – PR focus

Day 5: Push 2

- Delt, Triceps – Hypertrophy focus
- Chest – PR focus

Day 6: Off

Day 7: Legs 2

- Hams, Adductors, Glutes, Calves – Hypertrophy focus
- Quads – PR focus

Day 8: Pull 2

- Mid/Lower Back, Traps – Hypertrophy focus
- Lats, Rear Delts, Biceps – PR focus

Day 9: Off

Day 10: Repeat

Push 1

Core Movements – Perform each week

- **Sets in red are PR sets**

Incline Barbell Bench Press:

3 sets x 10-12 reps

- Take as many warm-ups as needed
- Each set should be to positive failure

Flat Dumbbell Bench:

3 sets x 8-10 reps

- Try to move up in weight when you can, but these are not PR sets—form should never suffer here

Seated Lateral Raises:

5 sets x 12-15 reps

- Pick a weight where 15 reps is positive failure for the first set.
- Resting minimally, make sure you get at least 12 reps each set.
- Adjust your rest times so that each set gets at least 12 reps with the same weight

Close Grip Bench:

2 sets 8-10 reps

- Try to hit PRs, but make sure your triceps are doing the work—not your chest
- There are many ways to get a PR here.
  - More total reps over the 2 sets

- More weight than the previous week (once you get to 2 sets of 10 reps, you will be forced to increase the weight)
- Less rest between sets

Seated Military Press:

1 set 10-12 reps

- Perform warm ups as needed
- This is a PR set--you must either get an additional rep or use more weight each time you cycle through

Overhead Rope Extensions:

3 set 15-20 reps

- These are done as a mechanical drop set. Start with hands separated. When you hit failure that way, keep hands separated on the eccentric, but put hands together (for leverage) on the positive portion. When you hit failure there, keep hands together the entire time and bang out a few extra partial reps. So, this is essentially a triple drop set

Pec Deck:

4 sets 20 reps

- Pure blood volume here—get blood in the area
- This is your hypertrophy day for chest, so push these HARD

Additional Movements – choose 1-2 movements per workout to supplement the volume of your PR body parts for the day.

- Learn to adjust these based on your soreness. This is NOT a hypertrophy day for triceps. If your triceps are getting very sore, then you should not be adding a movement here

Dips:
2 sets to failure

Clean and presses:
2 sets 12-15 reps (hang clean to press)

Replacement Movements – replace a core movement when you hit sticking point on PRs

Cable Crossovers:
4 sets 20 reps (as replacement for pec deck)

Incline Dumbbell Presses:
1 set x 8-10 reps (as flat barbell replacement)

Incline Barbell presses:
1 set x 8-10 reps (as flat barbell replacement)

Legs 1

Core Movements – Perform each week

- **Sets in red are PR sets**

Standing Calf (any variation):

4 sets x 15-20 reps

- Squeeze these—don't bounce. These aren't PR sets. Your goal is to contract the calf, not bounce up more weight

Seated Calf:

3 sets x 15-20 reps

- At the start of the movement, lean your body forward to place more weight over your feet. As the set gets harder, begin leaning back until you're actively pulling back on the handles to extend the set

Walking lunges:

3 sets 30 total steps (warm up)

Lying Leg curls:

1 set x 10-12 reps

- Add 1-2 forced reps, partial reps, and/or slow negative
- This is a PR set, not a hypertrophy set so make sure you're putting everything into this one set and getting stronger each week

Leg Press:
2-3 sets 10-20 reps (warm up)
3 sets of 20 reps

- These are hypertrophy sets so the focus in on FRYING the quads, not just pushing more weight. It's very easy to move up in weight here by tightening your knee wraps, widening your stance, not going as deep, etc. The goal is not to just use more weight—the goal is to make your quads sore.

Seated Leg Curls:
2 sets x 10-15 reps

- Your PR is the total reps with the same weight over the two sets (somewhere between 20-30 reps). A PR is more total reps than the previous workout

Leg extension – Barbell Squat super set:
3 sets of:
20 reps on leg extension
10 reps on squats

- These should be brutal. The leg extensions are to positive failure. The squat should follow IMMEDIATELY (within 10 seconds) of finishing the leg extensions

Adductor Machine:
1 set x 20 reps

- This is a PR set so get stronger each week

Additional Movements – choose 1-2 movements per workout to supplement the volume of your PR body parts for the day.

- Learn to adjust these based on your soreness. We have explained how more volume does not directly correlate to more growth. Your PR body parts on each day are for getting stronger—this is just a supplement to that. Do NOT just turn each body part into a hypertrophy-focused body part by adding volume to every PR-focused body part or you will stall progress.

Wide stance stiff leg deadlifts:
2-3 sets x 12-15 reps (a few reps short of failure)

Bulgarian split squats:
1 set x 20 reps per leg

Single Leg presses:
2 sets 15-20 reps

Hack Squats:
1 set 15-20 reps

Pull 1

Warm Up:

- Do a few sets of pull downs or cable pull overs to get blood in the lats and muscles around the shoulder.

Core Movements – Perform each week

- **Sets in red are PR sets**

Pull ups:

5 sets to failure

- Start with as few reps as you need to. If you're a larger bodybuilder who hasn't done pullups in a long time, you might be doing sets of 5 reps to start. That's fine.
- Whatever the total rep count is for a given workout, you must get more the next week.
  - E.g., if you get 25 total reps in the first workout, then 26 total reps in the next is a PR. It won't be very long until you're doing sets of 10+ reps—but only if you don't force the new reps. *Counting half reps as a PR is going to lead to a sticking point and stall progress.*

Deadlifts, Rack Pulls, or Pendlay Rows

Warm ups: as many as needed to get to your max weight

1 set x 5-8 reps

1 set x 10-12 reps

- Just like on squats, you have more than one movement to work with. If you're feeling strong on deads, always use those as the primary movement. If your legs are too sore from the leg workout, use rack deads as your back up movement.
- Pendlay rows are a deadlift/row hybrid. You start the exercise from the floor like a deadlift, and then turn it into a barbell row as you move through the movement.

Rope Pull Downs:
3 sets x 10-12 reps

- These are done with the rope attachment—the one you would typically use for triceps pushdowns. This is almost a hybrid pullover/pulldown movement. Adjust your form until you feel your lats being the prime mover. This is not a weight movement—the lats are a weak link in this position so you will need to be very focused on making sure they are pulling the rope handles down and not the other muscles of the back

Shrugs: (any variation)
3x15

- Work through these sets with minimal rest

One Arm Rows (Kroc Rows):
1 set x 15 reps

- These are done similarly to a standard one-arm row, but you will do them without a knee on a bench. You'll lean forward with your opposite hand on a bench or dumbbell rack. You will pronate your hands slightly so that the dumbbell is perpendicular to your torso (similarly to how your hand would be angled to hold a barbell in a barbell row). This allows for better leverages and heavier weight.

Reverse Pec Deck:

5 sets x 15 reps

Preacher Curls:

4 sets x 15-20 reps

- Form is everything here—these are not PR sets. These are to fry your biceps

Drag Curls:

3 sets x 10-12 reps

- There are many videos online of drag curl form— you basically just do a barbell curl while dragging the bar along your body

Additional Movements – choose 1-2 movements per workout to supplement the volume of your PR body parts for the day.

- Learn to adjust these based on your soreness.

Seated Rows:

3 sets x 10-15 reps

Hammer Strength pulldowns (any pulldown or row variation):
3 sets x 10-12

Cable curls (any variation):
6 sets 6 reps

- This is done one arm at a time—it's essentially one very long set where you rotate between arms for 6 sets of each arm. Only perform an additional bicep movement on EITHER the pull1 or pull 2 workouts—not both.

Push 2

Core Movements – Perform each week

- **Sets in red are PR sets**

Machine Press of your choice (typically a hammer press is best):

3 sets x 5-7 reps

- On the 3 sets of 5-7 reps, **you have multiple ways of achieving a PR**
  - *Increasing the total number of reps.* You can increase the total number of reps over the three sets. For example, if you did 3 sets of 5 reps with a weight this week for a total of 15 reps, then 1 set of 6 reps and 2 sets of 5 reps with the same weight the following week would be a 16 rep PR
  - *Increasing the weight.* Once you hit 7 reps in all three sets, you can increase the weight used
  - *Increasing the weight on the first set.* Increase the weight on the first set and then complete the second two sets with the same weight and reps as the previous week.

Incline Dumbbell Bench:

1 set x 6-8 reps
1 set x 10-12 reps

- These are PR sets, but form should not suffer. Keep yourself injury free, but get stronger each week

Cable Lateral Raises:

3 sets x 12-15 reps

Dead-Stop Skull Crushers on the Floor

3 sets x 10-12 reps

- Each rep should pause briefly on the floor, like in a deadlift

One Arm Behind-the-Neck Smith Machine Press

3 sets 10-12 reps

- This is performed on a traditional smith machine, but only one arm is used. The machine will still run smoothly along the bearings of each side—the arm being used does not need to be placed in the center of the bar

Dumbbell Front Raise:

3 sets 12-15 reps

- Don't swing these up. If you're not doing dumbbell shoulder press with 200lb dumbbells, you won't be able to contract your front delts to use more than about 70lb dumbbells here. If you're using more than that, you're swinging the weight and making it a trap movement

Machine Dips:

4 sets x 20 reps

Triceps Pushdowns:
3 sets x 10-15 reps

Additional Movements – choose 1-2 movements per workout to supplement the volume of your PR body parts for the day.

- Learn to adjust these based on your soreness. This is NOT a hypertrophy day for Chest. If your Chest is getting sore from this workout then you're not going to benefit from the hypertrophy work in the Push 1 session.

Dips:
2 sets to failure

Clean and presses:
2 sets 12-15 reps (hang clean to press)

Legs 2

Core Movements – Perform each week

- **Sets in red are PR sets**

Standing Calf (any variation):
3 sets x 15-20 reps

- Squeeze these—don't bounce. These aren't PR sets. Your goal is to contract the calf, not bounce up more weight

Seated Calf:
2-3 sets x 15-20 reps

Walking lunges:
3 sets 30 total steps (warm up)

Lying Leg curls:
4 sets x 10-12 reps

- Use as many warms-ups as needed. These are done to positive failure—not beyond that.

Squat (back squat or front squat – rotate between them as needed to always hit a PR):
1 set x 5-7 reps
1 set x 10-12 reps

- The goal is to get stronger every week, but ONLY if your form is unchanged. If you're putting the bar lower on your back, widening your stance, or resting 10 minutes in between sets to get a PR,

you're not getting stronger—you're just more
rested or have better leverage.

Dumbbell Leg curls:

3 sets x 10-12 reps

- Place a dumbbell between the soles of your feet.
  There are many videos online if you have trouble
  figuring the movement out.

Jefferson Squat:

4 sets x 15-20 reps

- This is an uncomfortable movement at first, but
  you'll understand why they're used as a
  hypertrophy movement when you're sore
  everywhere the next day.

Hack Squat:

1 set x 12-15 reps

- Use as many warm-ups as needed, but if you're not
  warm by this part of the workout, something is
  terribly wrong.
- Focus on getting stronger without any change in
  the movement.

***Additional Movements – choose 1 movement per
workout to supplement the volume of your PR body parts
for the day.***

- Quads are your PR movement for the day. It's very
  hard to get stronger on quads without also making
  them sore—so be very sure you truly need the
  additional workload before you add an additional

movement.

Bulgarian split squats:
1 set x 20 reps per leg

Single Leg presses:
2 sets 15-20 reps

Pull 2

Warm up:

- Perform a few sets of cable pull overs or light pulldowns to get the muscles of the back and shoulder properly warm and ready for the training session

Core Movements – Perform each week

- **Sets in red are PR sets**

Pull downs (overhand grip):

3 sets x 10-12 reps

- Focus on squeezing the lats. Pulldowns aren't a strength movement. Spread the scapula and then contract the lats. That is the goal here. If we can get stronger in that form—great. But don't sacrifice the contraction for weight.

Rack Pulls:

1 set x 5-7 reps
1 set x 10-12 reps

- Use as many warm-ups as necessary.
- I don't really care where you put the bar—it can be below the knee, at the knee, or even at the top of the knee. This isn't an ego lift and you don't get brownie points for putting the pins lower on your lower leg. This movement is to make your midback freakishly strong—so pick the pin location for that, not for internet points. I personally got the most

benefit from placing the bar at the top of my knee. Lower than that and I might have well just done a regular deadlift because the weights used would have been the same.

T-Bar Rows:

2-3 sets x 10-12 reps (not to failure)

1 set x 10-12 reps

- Keep some semblance of form but get f'n strong on these.

Way bent over rows:

3 sets x 10-12 reps

- Stand on a box if needed. These are bent over rows with a wider grip (a lot wider) where you stay bent over past parallel to the floor. You pull to the chest on these.

Barbell Curls:

1 Rest Pause set 15-20 total reps

- 1-2 warm up sets to get blood in the area and then right into the main set

Dumbbell Hammer Curls:

1 set 15-20 reps

- Straight set, not rest pause. Start with both arms at the same time. When you get close to failure, begin alternating arms for more momentum and leverage.

Rear Delt Dumbbell Swings:

2 sets x 12-15 reps

- Lay facing down on an incline bench and use dumbbells about twice as heavy as you would for standard bent over laterals. Keeping your arms straight, attempt to perform a rear lateral. You'll only be able to move the weight about 15 degrees---but that's the movement. Try to swing them out as far to the side as possible.

Additional Movements – choose 1-2 movements per workout to supplement the volume of your PR body parts for the day.

Hammer Strength pulldowns (any variation):
3 sets x 10-12

Hammer Strength Rows (any variation):
3 sets x 8-10 reps

Machine Curls (any variation):
6 sets x 6 reps

- Perform an additional bicep movement on EITHER pull 1 or pull 2, not both. This is meant to alternate between arms, so it would be essentially one very long set where you do 6 reps back and forth between arms.

Alternative Workouts

Phase 2

Push – Alternative

Core Movements – Perform each week

- **Sets in red are PR sets**

Incline Hammer Press:

1 set x 5-9 reps

1 set x 10-12 reps

- Take as many warm-ups as needed.
- Each set should be to positive failure.

Dumbbell Floor Presses:

3 sets x 8-10 reps

- Try to move up in weight when you can, but these are not PR sets—form should never suffer here.

Cable Lateral Raises:

3 sets x 12-15 reps

- Pick a weight where 15 reps is positive failure for the first set.
- Resting minimally, make sure you get at least 12 reps each set.
- Adjust your rest times so that each set gets at least 12 reps with the same weight.

Dumbbell Flys:

1 set x 20 reps

- This is in the style of a "widowmaker" from DC training.

Seated Military Press:

3 sets x 10-12 reps

Wide Grip Pushdowns:

1 set 15-20 reps

- Grab a lat pulldown bar and use it for pushdowns.
- Grab wider than shoulder width (slightly) and tuck your elbows into your side for the movement. You should feel a strong contraction in the long head of the triceps.

Close Grip Pushups:

4 sets x failure

- Pure blood volume here—get blood in the area.
- Rest as little as possible between sets.

Legs – Alternative

Core Movements – Perform each week

- **Sets in red are PR sets**

Standing Single Leg Calf Raise:

3 sets x 15-20 reps

- Grab a 25-35lb dumbbell and complete a set to failure while holding that dumbbell. As soon as you reach failure, drop the dumbbell and continue to failure again on the same leg.

Seated Calf:

2-3 sets x 15-20 reps

Single Leg Press:

3 sets x 12-15 reps

- Use as many warm up sets as necessary—these are essentially replacing the walking lunges as warm ups from Legs 1.

Seated Leg curls:

1 set x 9-11 reps
1 set x 14-19 reps

- Do NOT sacrifice form for a PR. It's not about just using more weight each week—it's about making your hamstrings smaller. They are a small muscle group and this is a single-joint movement. Because of this, the ultimate strength limit for the movement is rather low, so it will be slow progress for PRs if done correctly.

Favorite Leg Press or Hack Squat Machine

1 set x 5-7 reps
1 set x 10-12 reps

- If you have a specific machine that you really like where you train, then use that machine here.

Single Leg Curls:

3 sets x 10-12 reps

Jefferson Squats:

3 sets x 10-12 reps

- These are not PR sets. It is very difficult to use correct form on these with no weight, let alone with a new PR weight each week. Get the form correct and focus on contracting the correct muscles.

Adductor Machine:

1 set x 12-15 reps

- The adductor machine is one of those machines where you can very easily pile a ton of weight on with a few minor modifications to form. Do not fall down that path. The adductors are small muscles—if you're adding huge chunks of weight to the machine each week you can be sure that It's not because the relatively small muscles of the inner thigh got stronger and instead that you've just found a better mechanical advantage.

Pull - Alternative

Warm up:

- Perform a few sets of cable pull overs or light pulldowns to get the muscles of the back and shoulder properly warm and ready for the training session.

Core Movements – Perform each week

- **Sets in red are PR sets**

Favorite Lat Movement

4 sets x 10-12 reps

- If you have a favorite lat machine (pullover, hammer pulldown, etc) at your gym, this is the time to implement it.

Snatch Grip Deadlifts:

3 set x 7-9 reps

- Most of the "snatch grip" movements I see online are not a true snatch grip. Google "world record snatch" (careful that no kids are in the room…) and see what a snatch grip really is—your hands will be nearly to the collars.

Favorite Machine Row

2-3 sets x 10-12 reps (not to failure)

1 set x 10-12 reps

- If you have a favorite machine row at your gym— feel free to include it here.

Two Arm Dumbbell Rows:

3 sets x 10-12 reps

- These are done just like a regular barbell row, but with two dumbbells instead.

Barbell Spider Curls:

3 sets x 12-15 reps

Machine Curls

3 set 15-20 reps

- If you have a favorite bicep machine, feel free to use it here.

Reverse Cable Crossovers

3 sets x 15-20 reps

- Just grab the ball at the end of the cable—no need to use a handle attachment. The cables should be in the high position and you just do a reverse fly from there. There are many videos online if the exercise description is confusing.

Made in the USA
Middletown, DE
01 August 2023

36110995R00033